Air Fryer Coc

*How to Cook Beautiful and Yummy
Recipes to become like a Michelin
Star Chef using your Air Fryer*

SABRINA BRADLEY

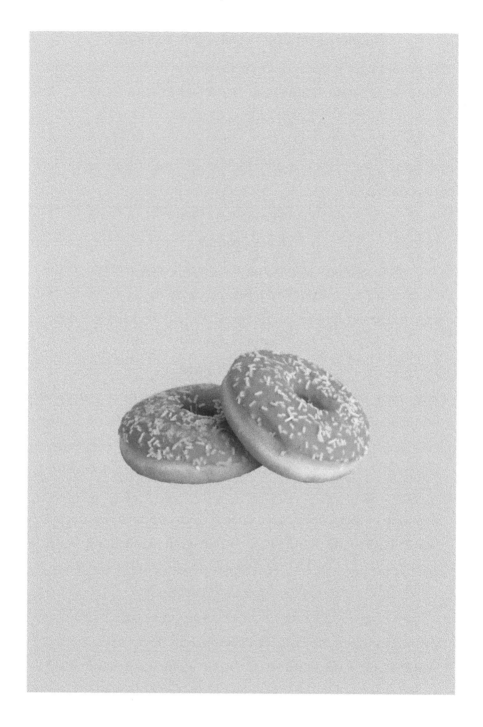

Table of Contents

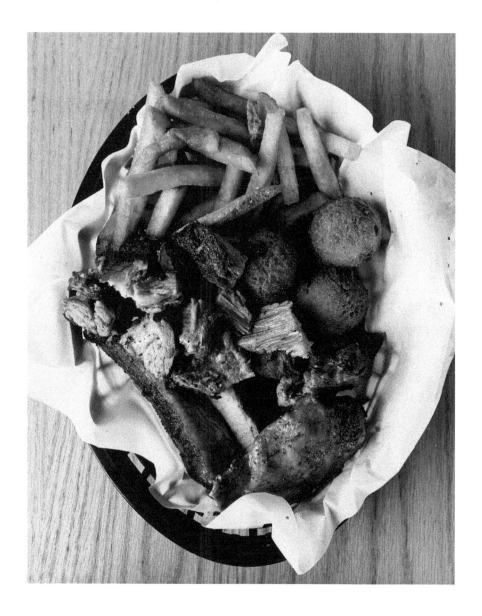

Introduction

Now a days an Air fryer is a must have kitchen gadget because of its healthy cooking process. This machine uses air as a medium to transfer heat to your food hence you do not need any excess number of oils to cook the food. Conventionally people use boiled food to avoid the use of oil but many people don't like the taste of boiled food also not every food can be boiled.

Thanks to Air fryer now you can enjoy almost every recipe you love. Air fryer can cook almost everything for you. Just follow the proper steps and give yourself some relaxing time rest of things will be done automatically.

Keeping in view the benefits and ease of cooking in an air fryer we have developed a book for our reader that help the readers to understand how to use this machine properly, not only this, the book contains hundreds of unique recipes you can follow and easily make in your air fryer.

Now you don't need to compromise on your favorite recipes just bring in the air fryer and enjoy the food you love without compromising your health.

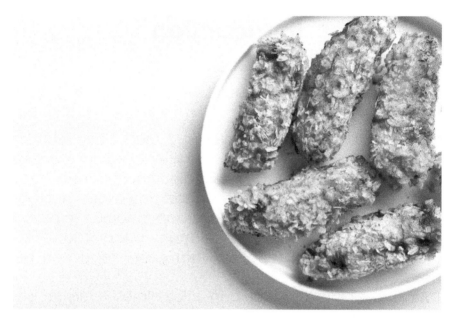

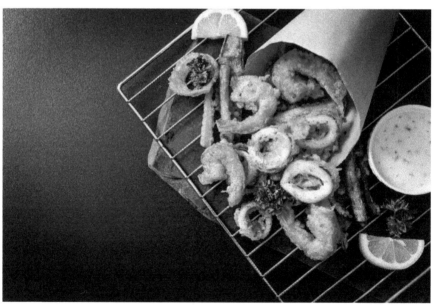

CHAPTER 1:

How to setup the Air-Fryer?

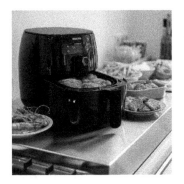

What Is an Air Fryer?

An air fryer is basically a kitchen gadget that can be used to cook various food items, there are so many brands available in the market but the basic function in all of them is same that is cooking food through hot air, these machines work just like ovens to cook the food. However, the texture of cooked food in an air fryer is somehow different than the food which is cooked in an oven.

Setting up An Air Fryer

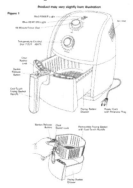

As we mentioned earlier there are various brands available for air fryers in the market and one can easily buy them and start using them out of the box. Just follow the directions given in their manual.

Because all the air fryers have same function for cooking the food so we have developed some general guidelines that can be followed to setup your air fryer.

- Take out your air fryer out of the box and remove any adhesive martials (scotch tape and other) that may be used by manufacturer to keep the things in place.

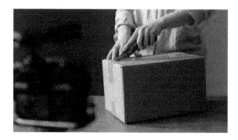

- Place your machine on a flat and dry place, as this machine produces heat so you must select a heat proof surface for placing this machine.
- Find out the power cod and make sure that you have a suitable power outlet available to power up your machine.

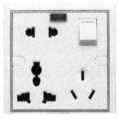

- Almost every model comes with a frying basket, just firmly grasp the drawer containing that basket to take out that basket out of your machine.

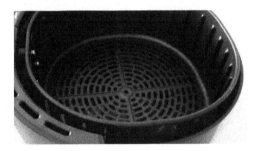

- Now close the drawer leaving the basket outside and power on the machine. Just wash the basket with running water to make it ready for later use.

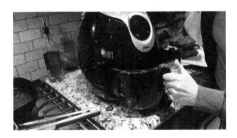

- Just set the temperature to normal range and run the machine without placing any food in it for few minutes. This is important because upon 1st use the machine will produces some odors that you don't want to be mixed with your loved foods.

- Now after running it or few minutes turn off your device.
- Now your air fryer is ready to be used for cooking your favorite foods.

General Guidelines to Use an Air Fryer

- Always put your food in the air fryer basket.

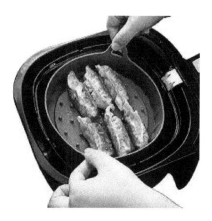

- It is recommended to never fully cover the basket with your food as it will block the air flow and your food will not be cooked properly, as general rule always fill the basket to 2/3 portion.

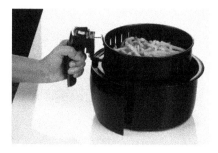

- After putting your food in the basket make sure that you have properly placed the basket in its place and the drawer is completely closed there should be no extra space between the drawer and your machine.

- Select the temperature from the dialing knob or button given on your machine.

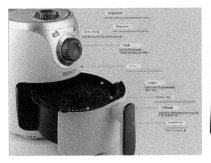 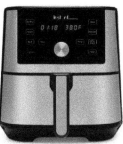

- Similarly set the time for cooking by adjusting the temperature settings. Note you can adjust the time according to situation because most of the recipes provide general timing guidelines and depending upon the environment conditions and other factor the time may vary so adjust the time according to your own requirements.
- Once the power and heat light come on your machine is now in working mode. Be careful to handle the machine at this stage because it will be hot.

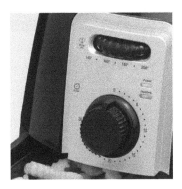

- Always use the grate provided with air fryer in case your model does not have the one then buys that for you, it allows even cooking of food because of good air flow.

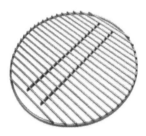

- Never open the drawer while heat light is on, the machine light will come on and off during the cooking process. When the temperature is maintained the light will goes off and comes again once the temperature is dropped, once the lights go off, open the drawer and Shake the basket of the air fryer while cooking the food it will help to cook food properly. But never open the drawer when "HEAT light is ON"

- Once the cooking time is finished allow the food to rest inside for 15 seconds to let the heat and steam comes out.
- Extreme caution must be followed while handling the machine because it involves heating. Use a pair of gloves to handle the basket while taking out your food.

CHAPTER 2:

Meat Recipes

We have included several meat recipes in this chapter of this book to enjoy your meals without compromising your meat intake.

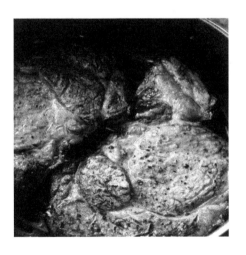

1. Steak With Mushroom And Black Pepper

Preparation Time: 60min | Serving: 4 | Difficulty: Easy

Nutritional Info: Calories: 275kcal | Fat: 16g | Carb: 7g | Protien: 25g

Ingredients

- Ribeye steak, 1 pound Cornstarch, 1 teaspoon
- Rice wine, 1 tablespoon Lime juice, 1 tablespoon
- Soy sauce, 2 teaspoons
- Grated ginger, 2 tablespoons
- Black pepper, 1/4 teaspoon

Sauce ingredients:

- Mushrooms thinly sliced, 8
- Garlic finely chopped, 1 tablespoon
- Oyster sauce, 1 tablespoon

Steps for preparation

1. Combine all the ingredients inside a Ziplock bag and then marinate for around 2 hours.

2. Line the fry basket with aluminum foil.

3. Place the steak within the Air fryer's basket and then air fry at 350F for 12 minutes. In the middle of the cooking process, add whole components into the steak and then stir well. Air Fry again for 5 minutes.

4. Carefully add the sauce ingredients to a skillet and Stir continuously till the sauce thickens.

5. Put the steak cubes inside the sauce and cover with the remaining sauce.

2. Stuffed Zucchini Asian Meatball

Preparation Time: 15min | Serving: 4 | Difficulty: Easy

Nutritional Info: Calories: 221kcal | Fat: 16g | Carb: 4g | Protien: 15g

Ingredients

- Ground beef, 1 pound

- Beaten, 1 egg

- Minced onion, 1/4 cup

- Chopped basil, 2 tablespoons

- Oyster sauce, 2 tablespoons

- Corn starch, 1 teaspoon

- Black pepper, 1/4 teaspoon

- Zucchinis peeled, 2 larges

Steps for preparation

1. Combine all the ingredients, except the zucchini, in a medium-size bowl, then marinate at room temperature for about 15 minutes.

2. Line Air fryer's basket with a big sheet of aluminum and drizzle some oil.

3. Round the zucchini into one-inch pieces and hollow the middle using a sharp knife. Afterward, add the beef combination to the zucchini and place it inside the fryer basket without spilling.

4. Air fry at 375F for 10 minutes and apply some oil at the end of the cooking process.

3.   Roasted Tri-Tip

Preparation Time: 60min | Serving: 2 | Difficulty: Easy

Nutritional Info: Calories: 323kcal | Fat: 21g | Carb: 1g | Protien: 31g

Ingredients

- Tri-tip roast, 2 pounds

- Garlic, 6-8 cloves

- Olive oil, 1/4 cup

- Salt, 2 1/2 teaspoon

- Garlic powder, 1 teaspoon

- Black pepper, 1/2 teaspoon

Steps for preparation

1. Blend the seasoning ingredients in a blender.

2. Now wash the tri-tip then dry with a paper towel then place it inside a large Ziplock bag.

3. Place the seasoning mixture within the bag, compress as much air as possible, and close the bag. Spread the spices and rub the beef with them;

make sure that all areas are coated with the paste. Leave it at room temperature for around 2 hours.

4. Now air fry at 400 F for around 25 minutes before the meat's target internal temperature is achieved, 160F.

5. Now let the roast left about ten minutes before taking it out of the air fryer.

4. Beef Empanadas Pie Crust

Preparation Time: 30min | Serving: 4 | Difficulty: Easy

Nutritional Info: Calories: 545kcal | Fat: 37g | Carb: 30g | Protien: 22g

Ingredients

- Ground beef, 1 pound Pickled jalapeno, 1-2 tablespoon Corn starch, 1 teaspoon

- Cumin, 1 teaspoon Chili powder, 1 teaspoon

- Salt, 1/4 teaspoon Pepper, 1/4 teaspoon

- Olive oil, 1 teaspoon Minced garlic, 2 tablespoons

- Diced onions, 1/4 cup Pie crust thawed, 2 rolls

- Mexican blend cheese, 1 cup

- Beaten, 1 egg

Steps for preparation

1. In a big bowl, combine ground beef and jalapeno, corn starch, and cumin, add chili powder with salt and pepper, and leave for around 5 to 5 minutes.

2. Line the air fryer's basket with a barbecue pad.

3. In a big pan, sauté the garlic and the onion for around 2 minutes till fragrant. Add ground beef, then whisk till the beef is cooked through and the onion is translucent.

4. Then Roll out those pie crusts. Combine the left side of the pie by using a rolling pin to roll it out. Repeat the step above and get some circular crusts as required.

5. Place the circular parts of the pie crust at the counter and place the desired quantity of filling and cheese in the middle. Fold these pie crust in half and keep these fillings inside.

6. Carefully pass the empanadas towards the fryer's basket. Brush the upper surface with the egg and air fry for 7 minutes at 350F. Now change the sides and again cook for 2 minutes till golden brown.

5.   Gochujang Mayo With Meatballs

Preparation Time: 15min | Serving: 4 | Difficulty: Easy

Nutritional Info: Calories: 378kcal | Fat: 29g | Carb: 7g | Protien: 21g

Ingredients

- Boiled beef 1 pound

- Onion finely chopped, 1/4 cup

- Soy sauce, 2 Tablespoon

- Corn starch, 2 teaspoons Dried basil, 1 teaspoon

- Garlic powder, 1 teaspoon

- Onion powder, 1 teaspoon

- White pepper powder, 1/4 teaspoon

Ingredients for sauce:

- Gochujang, 1 teaspoon

- Mayonnaise, 2 Tablespoon Mirin, 2 Tablespoon

Steps for preparation

1. Line an air-fried basket with a barbecue pad or a sheet thinly coated with cooking oil.

2. Combine all the ingredients of the meatball and mold them into around 1-inch balls. Put some oil in the meatballs, and then air fry at 350F for 8 to 10 minutes.

3. Meanwhile, take a small bowl and combine all the components of the sauce.

4. Dip these meatballs in the mayonnaise to serve when fully cooked.

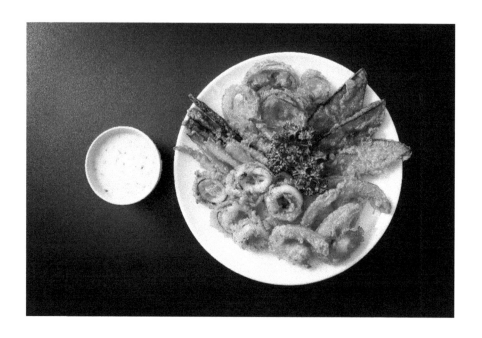

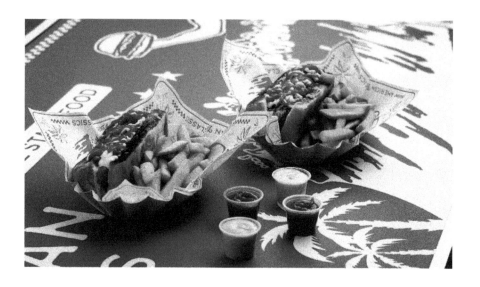

CHAPTER 3:

Fish and Seafood

This chapter is intended to enlist easy to make recipes for seafood lovers. We have mentioned the recipes which are easy to make, and you can prepare them in the least time.

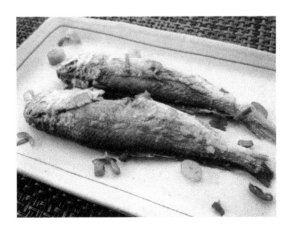

6.   Salmon Foil Packet

Preparation Time:10min | Serving: 4 | Difficulty: Easy

Nutritional   Info: Calories:245kcal | Fat: 8g | Carb:
19g | Protien: 26g

Ingredients

- Salmon fillets, 4-4-ounce, 1 lb.

- Green beans, 4 cups

- Sodium soy sauce, 4 tablespoons

- Honey, 2 tablespoons

- Sesame seeds, 2 teaspoons

- Garlic powder, 1 teaspoon

- Ginger powder, ½ teaspoon

- Kosher salt, ½ teaspoon

- White pepper, ¼ teaspoon

- Kosher salt Canola oil spray

Steps for preparation

1. In a mixing cup, whisk all ingredients the soy sauce,
   the honey,   the canola   oil,   the sesame   seeds,

the garlic and the ginger powder, and then red pepper flakes.

2. Now Place the 4 layers of 12" x 11" foil over the baking sheet. Spray fillets and then green beans with a cooking spray and then season to taste with the salt. Divide and then center the green beans sliced between the foil sheet. Put salmon fillet on top of green beans.

3. Pour sauce over each slice of fish and close the foil firmly.

4. Place the closely packed packets in the air fryer. Turn the 390-degree unit or use fish steering on certain models. Set the time to 12 mins. Rest for around 5 mins before opening the packets

7. Blackened Shrimp In Air Fryer

Preparation Time:5min | Serving: 4 | Difficulty: Easy

Nutritional Info: Calories:175kcal | Fat: 9g | Carb: 5g | Protien: 23g

Ingredients

- Large shrimp, 1 pound
- Olive oil, 2 tablespoons
- Blackened seasoning, 1 tablespoon
- Favorite dipping sauce
- Lemon wedges
- Parsley, chopped

Steps for preparation

1. Preheat air fryer at about 400 degrees for about 5 mins.

2. In the mixing bowl, add shrimp and olive oil, then draining out any excess in the bottom.

3. Toss shrimp with the blackened seasonings.

4. When hot, gently oil the air fryer basket. Then Add some shrimp.

5. Cook at about 400 degrees for 5 to 6 mins, shaking halfway through. Now Cook before the shrimp is done, turn pink and curl.

6. Remove and then serve with your dip sauce.

8. Spicy Marmalade Sauce With Coconut Shrimps

Preparation Time: 8min | Serving: 2 | Difficulty: Easy

Nutritional Info: Calories: 486kcal | Fat: 18g | Carb: 50g | Protien: 32g

Ingredients

- Shrimp, 1 lb.

- All-purpose flour, 1/2 cup

- Cayenne pepper, 1/2 teaspoon

- Kosher salt, 1/4 teaspoon

- Fresh ground pepper, 1/4 teaspoon

- Panko bread, 1/2 cup

- Coconut milk, 8 ounces Egg, 1

- Shredded, sweetened coconut, 1/2 cup

for the sauce:

- Orange marmalade, 1/2 cup

- Honey, 1 tablespoon

- Mustard, 1 teaspoon

- Hot sauce, 1/4 teaspoon

Steps for preparation

1. Set aside all the shrimps after rinsing them.

2. Combine the rice, salt, vinegar, cayenne pepper, and panko bread crumbs in a mixing bowl. Place aside.

3. In a shallow mixing cup, add coconut milk and the egg. Place aside. Shred coconut into a third shallow bowl.

4. Dip all the shrimps one at a time in a flour mixture, then in coconut oil, and eventually in coconut.

5. Heat air fryer to 400°F. Put the shrimps in the basket. Bake for about 10 -12 mins, or till all shrimps are golden and cooked through.

6. When all the shrimps are frying, combine the marmalade, sugar, vinegar, and the hot sauce in a mixing bowl.

7. Serve the shrimps directly with the sauce.

9.   Crispy Fish Air Fried

Preparation Time: 8min | Serving: 3 | Difficulty: Easy

Nutritional Info: Calories: 201kcal | Fat: 3g | Carb: 5g | Protien: 32g

Ingredients

- Cod, 1 lb.

- Sea salt

- Gluten-free flour, 2 tablespoons

- Eggs, 2

- Gluten-free panko, 1/2 cup

- Onion powder, 1 tablespoon

- Fresh dill, minced, 1 tablespoon

- Dry mustard, ½ tablespoon

- Paprika, ½ tablespoon

- Lemon zest, packed, ½ tablespoon

For the Yogurt Dip:

- Non-fat yogurt, 1/2 Cup

- Fresh lemon juice, 2 tablespoons

- Fresh dill, minced, 1 tablespoon

- Sea salt, to taste

Steps for preparation

1. Preheat air fryer to 400F and coat mesh basket with the cooking spray.

2. Pat cod dry with a paper towel and season generously with salt. Fill a big, rimmed plate halfway with flour. In a big mixing cup, thoroughly beat eggs. Then, in a big bowl, combine panko and remaining fish ingredients and swirl till well combined.

3. Coat cod parts in flour, then into egg mixture, using one side. Check that fish is covered in the egg but not dripping with it. And wrap it in panko. Coat fish in panko with the hand and put it in an air fryer basket. Repeat for the remaining items, leaving a little gap between them in the basket.

4. Coat tops with the cooking spray. Flip softly and simmer for another 8-10 mins. Finally, if the fish's underside has lost any crispness, turn it again and simmer for another 2-3 mins.

5. When the fish is frying, mix all of the ingredients and season with the salt to taste.

6. Serve the fish alongside the dip.

10.   Cajun Shrimps Dinner In Air Fryer

Preparation Time: 10min | Serving: 2 | Difficulty: Easy

Nutritional Info: Calories: 284kcal | Fat: 14g | Carb: 8g | Protien: 31g

Ingredients

- Cajun, 1 tablespoon
- Jumbo shrimp, 24
- Andouille sausage, 6 ounces
- Zucchini, 8 ounces
- Yellow squash, 8 ounces
- Red bell pepper, 1
- Kosher salt, 1/4 teaspoon
- Olive oil, 2 tablespoons

Steps for preparation

1. Toss all shrimps with Cajun spices in a mixing bowl.
2. Toss with oil, bacon, zucchini, squash, bell peppers, and salt.
3. Preheat air fryer to 400F.

4. Move all the shrimps and vegetables to air fryer and cook for 8 mins, shaking basket 2-3 times.

5. Set aside and then repeat with the remaining shrimps and vegetables.

6. Transfer the first batch to the air fryer and cook for 1 minute after the second batch has finished cooking.

11.   Parmesan Shrimps In Air Fryer

Preparation Time: 8min | Serving: 2 | Difficulty: Easy

Nutritional   Info: Calories: 130kcal | Fat: 4g | Carb:

15g | Protien: 4g

Ingredients

- Peeled shrimp, 2 pounds

- Cloves Garlic, minced, 4

- Parmesan cheese, grated, 2/3 cup

- Pepper, 1 teaspoon

- Oregano, 1/2 teaspoon

- Basil, 1 teaspoon

- Onion powder, 1 teaspoon

- Olive oil, 2 tablespoons

- Lemon, quartered

Steps for preparation

1. In a large bowl, combine garlic, parmesan cheese, pepper, oregano, basil, onion powder and olive oil.

2. Gently toss shrimp in mixture until evenly-coated.

3. Spray air fryer basket with non-stick spray and place shrimp in a basket.

4. Cook at 350 degrees for 8-10 minutes or until seasoning on shrimp is browned.

5. Squeeze the lemon over the shrimp before serving.

12. Sandwich Of Fish Finger

Preparation Time: 6min | Serving: 2 | Difficulty: Easy

Nutritional Info: Calories: 205kcal | Fat: 3g | Carb: 4g | Protien: 23g

Ingredients

- Small cod fillets, 4
- Salt, to taste
- Pepper, to taste
- Flour, 2 tablespoons
- Dried breadcrumbs, 40g
- Spray oil
- Frounceen peas, 250g
- Greek yogurt, 1 tablespoon
- 10–12 capers
- Lemon juice
- Bread rolls, 4

Steps for preparation

1. Pre-heat the Air Fryer.

2. Take each of the cod fillets, season with salt and pepper and lightly dust in the flour. Then roll quickly in the breadcrumbs. The idea is to get a light coating of breadcrumbs on the fish rather than a thick layer. Repeat with each cod fillet.

3. Add a few sprays of oil spray to the bottom of the fryer basket. Place the cod fillets on top and cook on the fish setting (200c) for 15 mins.

4. While the fish is cooking, cook the peas in boiling water for a couple of minutes on the hob or the microwave. Drain and then add to a blender with the creme fraiche, capers and lemon juice to taste. Blitz until combined.

5. Once the fish has cooked, remove it from the Air Fryer and start layering your sandwich with the bread, fish and pea puree.

13.   Crabs Air Fried

Preparation Time: 10min | Serving: 2 | Difficulty: Easy

Nutritional Info: Calories: 105kcal | Fat: 1g | Carb: 2g | Protien: 21g

Ingredients

- Large eggs, 2 Mayonnaise, 2 tablespoons

- Dijon mustard, 1 teaspoon

- Worcestershire sauce, 1 teaspoon

- Old bay seasoning, 1 ½ teaspoon

- Fresh pepper to taste

- Green onion, ¼ cup

- Lump crab meat, 1 pound

- Panko, ⅓ to ½ cup

Steps for preparation

1. Combine the egg, mayonnaise, Dijon mustard, Worcestershire, Old Bay in a medium bowl and mix well. Add the finely chopped green onion to the mayonnaise mixture and mix gently.

2. Add the crab to the mayonnaise mix until all incorporated. Add the panko to the crab/mayonnaise mix and fold together until just combined. Be careful not to over-mix while keeping the crab chunks intact.

3. Cover the crab mix and place it in the refrigerator for approximately 1 hour.

4. Shape into approximately 8 crab rounds of 1 inch thick. Make sure to not pack the cakes too tightly.

5. Preheat the air-fryer to 350F. Once the air-fryer reaches the desired temperature, gently place 4 crab rounds into the basket and set to air fry for 10 minutes. The crab cake should be set and with a light crust. Make sure to flip the crab cakes after 5 minutes to accomplish even cooking.

6. When ready, gently transfer to a plate. Serve with a lemon wedge

14.   Crusted Salmon Garlic Parmesan

Preparation Time: 5min | Serving: 2 | Difficulty: Easy

Nutritional Info: Calories: 530kcal | Fat: 28g | Carb: 11g | Protien: 45g

Ingredients

- Salmon, 1 lb.

- Black pepper, ¼ tablespoon

- Plain breadcrumbs, 1/4 cup

- Shredded parmesan cheese, 1/4 cup

- Italian seasoning, 1/2 teaspoon

- Unsalted butter melted, 2 tablespoons

- Minced garlic, 2 teaspoons

Steps for preparation

1. Start by preheating the Air fryer to 400 degrees F. Line baking sheet with parchment paper or aluminum foil, spray the basket with cooking spray.

2. Place salmon on a prepared baking sheet, skin side down. Pat dry with a paper towel.

3. In a medium mixing bowl, combine breadcrumbs (or Panko), Parmesan cheese and Italian seasoning. In another bowl, melt butter. Add garlic and stir. Add to the breadcrumb mixture. Stir well.

4. Season salmon with black pepper (no need for salt since Parmesan is pretty salty already). Divide the crust mixture evenly on top of each salmon piece, gently pressing onto the fish.

5. Set temperature to 400 degrees F, let it preheat for 4 minutes. Place salmon with crust, skin side down, in the basket and bake. Check the internal temperature to make sure the fish is done. If you are also roasting a vegetable side dish in the air fryer, you can add the salmon to cook in the same basket in the last 10 minutes. That way, everything will be done at the same time!

6. Serve immediately with vegetable side dishes

15. Southern Fried Catfish In Air Fryer

Preparation Time: 12min | Serving: 2 | Difficulty: Easy

Nutritional Info: Calories: 391kcal | Fat: 11g | Carb: 28g | Protien: 44g

Ingredients

- Catfish Fillets, 2 pounds
- Milk, 1 cup Lemon, 1
- Yellow Mustard, 1/2 cup

Cornmeal Seasoning Mix

- Cornmeal, 1/2 cup All-purpose flour, 1/4 cup
- Dried parsley flakes, 2 tablespoons
- Kosher salt, 1/2 teaspoon Black pepper, 1/4 teaspoon Chili powder, 1/4 teaspoon
- Garlic powder, 1/4 teaspoon
- Granulated onion powder, 1/4 teaspoon
- Cayenne pepper, 1/4 teaspoon

Steps for preparation

1. Place Catfish into a flat container and add Milk.

2. Cut Lemon in half and squeeze about two teaspoons of juice into Milk to make Buttermilk.

3. Place the container in the refrigerator and let Fillets soak for 15 minutes.

4. In a shallow bowl, combine Cornmeal Seasoning Ingredients.

5. Remove Fillets from Buttermilk and pat dry with paper towels.

6. Spread Mustard generously over both sides of Fillets.

7. Dip each Fillet into a Cornmeal mixture and coat well to make a thick coating.

8. Place Fillets into greased Air Fryer Basket. Spray generously with oil.

9. Cook at 390/400 degrees for 10 minutes. Flip over Fillets and spray with oil and cook for an additional 3-5 minutes.

16. Salmon Croquettes In Air Fryer

Preparation Time: 20min | Serving: 4 | Difficulty: Medium

Nutritional Info: Calories: 154kcal | Fat: 8g | Carb: 3g | Protien: 18g

Ingredients

- Pink salmon bones, 29.5-ounce

- Medium carrots grated, 1

- Brown onion grated, 1

- Large eggs, 2

- Mayonnaise, 1/4 cup

- Matzo meal, 2 tablespoons

- Chives chopped, 1 tablespoon

- Italian seasoning blend, 2 teaspoons

- Lemon juice, 2 teaspoons

- Kosher salt, 1 teaspoonBlack pepper, 1/4 teaspoon

Steps for preparation

1. Mix Aioli and place in an airtight container in the refrigerator.

2. Remove skin and bones from Salmon and place into a medium bowl.

3. Peel and grate carrot and place into the bowl with salmon.

4. Grate the onion and squeeze out excess water and add to bowl with salmon.

5. Add eggs, mayonnaise, matzo meal, Italian seasonings, chives, lemon juice, salt, pepper and mix together well.

6. Form into 12 sections and roll into balls.

7. Flatten out balls onto a cookie sheet to be about 3 inches diameter by 3/4 inches thick.

8. Place patties into the refrigerator for 30 minutes.

9. Place 6 patties in a single layer into greased air fryer basket and spray well with oil.

10. Cook at 400 degrees for 6 minutes and then flip over.

11. Spray again with oil and cook for 4 minutes, or until brown on both sides.

12. Garnish with chives and lemon zest. Serve with Lemon Dill Aioli

17. Lemon Garlic Shrimp, Air Fryer

Preparation Time: 8min | Serving: 2 | Difficulty: Easy

Nutritional Info: Calories: 129kcal | Fat: 3g | Carb: 14g | Protien: 3g

Ingredients

- Small shrimp, 1-pound

- Olive oil, 1 Tablespoon

- Garlic cloves, minced, 4

- Lemon, juice, 1

- Parsley, chopped, 1/4 cup

- Sea salt, 1/4 teaspoon

Steps for preparation

1. Heat your air fryer to 400°F.

2. In a bowl, combine the shrimp, olive oil, garlic, salt, lemon zest, and red pepper flakes (if using). Toss to coat.

3. Transfer the shrimp to the basket of your fryer. Cook for 5-8 minutes, shaking the basket halfway through or until the shrimp are cooked through.

4. Pour the shrimp into a serving bowl and toss with lemon juice and parsley. Season with additional salt to taste.

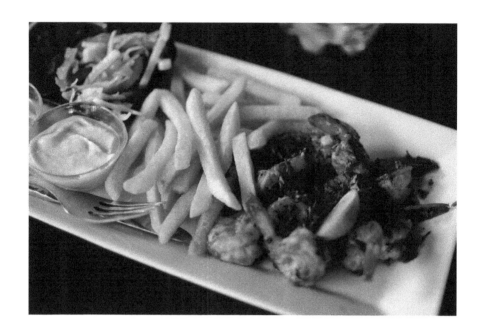

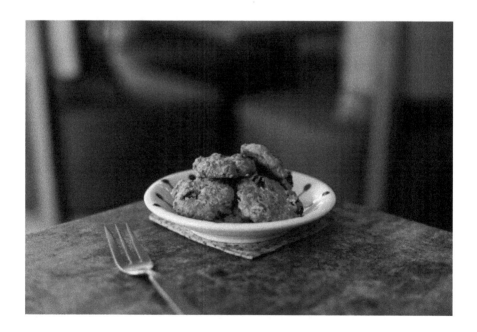

CHAPTER 4:

Vegetable and Side Recipes

D o you love veg food and get bored with meat recipes? Don't worry; we have a huge list of vegetable recipes in this chapter; these recipes are easy to make, but these are healthy.

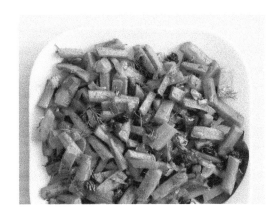

18.   Air-Fried Cheesy Potatoes

Preparation Time: 10min | Serving: 6 | Difficulty: Easy

Nutritional   Info: Calories: 137kcal | Fat: 3g | Carb: 22g | Protien: 5g

Ingredients

- Russet potatoes, 4

- Reduced-fat milk, 1 cup

- All-purpose flour, 2 tablespoons

- cheddar cheese, ½ cup

- Coarsely chopped, 1 cup

- Kosher salt, ¼ teaspoon

- Cayenne pepper, ¼ teaspoon

Steps for preparation

1. Pierce the potatoes all over with the fork.

2. In meanwhile, heat the 3/4 cup milk into the small saucepan to boil over medium-high heat. Whisk remaining 1/4 cup of milk and the flour in a small bowl until smooth. Now Bring to a simmer, still

whisking. Remove from the heat. Reserve the 2 tablespoons of cheddar. Stir remaining cheddar in the pan till blended and smooth.

3. Slice the potatoes into half; gently mash inside of every potato until it is loose and crumbly. Then layer 4 half of the potatoes at a time into the air fryer basket. Divide the 1 tablespoon of cheddar between potatoes.

4. Cook potatoes at 350°F till cheese is melted and potato skins are crisp around 5 mins.

5. Top potatoes with the chives, and serve.

19. Air-Fried Vegetable Medley

Preparation Time: 20min | Serving: 4 | Difficulty: Easy

Nutritional Info: Calories: 116kcal | Fat: 7g | Carb: 13g | Protien: 2g

Ingredients

- Small eggplant, ½ cup
- Small zucchini, 1
- Summer squash, (1 cup)
- Shiitake mushrooms, 1 cup
- Grape tomatoes, 1 cup
- Olive oil, 2 tablespoons
- Garlic cloves, 2
- Dried oregano, ½ teaspoon
- Kosher salt, ½ teaspoon Lemon zest, 1 teaspoon

Steps for preparation

1. In a big cup, mix eggplant, courgettis, summer squash, mushrooms, onions, olive oil, garlic, oregano and salt.

2. Cook vegetables into air fryer with the even layer at about 360°F for about 10 mins, stirring halfway through, till tender and the sides are golden brown.

3. Now Keep the cooked vegetables warm in a 200°F oven when cooking. Sprinkle with the lemon zest before serving.

20. Ginger With Shishito Peppers

Preparation Time: 10min | Serving: 4 | Difficulty: Easy

Nutritional Info: Calories: 34kcal | Fat: 2g | Carb: 5g | Protien: 1g

Ingredients

- Shishito peppers, 2 Oil, 1 teaspoon

- Soy sauce, 1 tablespoon

- Lime juice, 1 tablespoon

- Honey, 1 teaspoon

- Grated ginger, ½ teaspoon

Steps for preparation

1. Toss the peppers with the oil in a medium cup.

2. Put the peppers in the air fryer basket. Now cook at about 390°F for 6 to 7 mins or till blistered and tender, meanwhile shake the basket.

3. In the same medium cup, mix soy sauce, lime juice, honey and ginger. Add the cooked pepper and then toss to coat properly.

21. Roasted Vegetables In The Air Fryer

Preparation Time: 10min | Serving: 4 | Difficulty: Easy

Nutritional Info: Calories: 39kcal | Fat: 2g | Carb: 4g | Protien: 1g

Ingredients

- tender vegetables (zucchini, summer squash, pepper, baby mushrooms, cauliflower head, asparagus) or firm vegetables (baby potato, carrot, turnip, summer squash, celeriac), make cubes, 3 cups

- vegetable oil, 2 teaspoons

- salt, ¼ teaspoon

- black pepper, ¼ teaspoon

- Seasoning, ¼ teaspoon

- The dipping sauce, as per need

Steps for preparation

1. Preheat the air fryer to about 360°F. Add vegetables, oil, a pinch of salt, pepper and the

desired seasoning to the cup. Toss to coat evenly;

put in air fryer basket.

2. Cook the tender vegetables for 10 minutes, stirring

for 5 mins. Cook the firm vegetables for 15 minutes,

stirring after 5 mins. Serve with the dipping sauce.

22. Mexican-Style Air-Fried Corn

Preparation Time: 10min | Serving: 4 | Difficulty: Easy

Nutritional Info: Calories: 20kcal | Fat: 7g | Carb: 35g | Protien: 6g

Ingredients

- Ear corn, 4

- Cooking spray, as per need

- Unsalted butter, 1½ tablespoons

- Chopped garlic, 2 teaspoons

- Lime zest plus, 1 tablespoon

- Kosher salt, ½ teaspoon

- Black pepper, ½ teaspoon

- Chopped cilantro, 2 tablespoons

Steps for preparation

1. Lightly coat the corn with the cooking spray and put it into an air fryer basket in a single layer. Now Cook at about 400°F until soft and finely charred for

14 mins, turning the corn halfway through the cooking process.

2. Meanwhile, combine butter, garlic, the lime zest and juice of a lime in a shallow microwave bowl. And then Microwave on HIGH till butter is melted, the garlic is fragrant for around 30 seconds. Put the corn on a plate and pour over the butter mixture. Now Sprinkle with salt and pepper, and cilantro. Serve it.

23.   Kale Chips Air Fried

Preparation Time: 5min | Serving: 2 | Difficulty: Easy

Nutritional Info: Calories: 40kcal | Fat: 9g |

Ingredients

- Packed kale leaves, 6 cups Olive oil, 1 tablespoon

- Soy sauce, 1½ teaspoons Salt, 1teaspoon

- Sesame seeds (white), ½ teaspoon

- Ground cumin, ¼ teaspoon

Steps for preparation

1. Coat the air-fryer with the cooking spray.

2. In a medium cup, combine kale with oil and the soya sauce and salt; rub leaves together to be fully covered.In your air fryer basket, put the kale mixture. Now Coat the leaves with the cooking spray. And Cook at 375°F in air fryer till crispy, 10-12 mins, shaking basket and stirring leaves every 3 to 4 mins. Remove from basket and sprinkle some sesame seeds with cumin.

24. Balsamic Glazed Carrots Air-Fried

Preparation Time: 10min | Serving: 2 | Difficulty: Easy

Nutritional Info: Calories: 35kcal | Fat: 2g | Carb: 4g | Protien: 1g

Ingredients

- Olive oil, 1 tablespoon

- Honey, 1 teaspoon

- Kosher salt, ¼ teaspoon

- Black pepper, ¼ teaspoon

- Baby carrots, 1 pound

- Balsamic glaze, 1 tablespoon

- Butter, 1 tablespoon

- Chopped chives, 2 teaspoons

Steps for preparation

1. Preheat the air fryer to about 390°F. Coat the air fryer basket with the cooking spray. In a big cup, combine the olive oil, sugar, salt and pepper.

2. Now Add carrots and then toss to coat evenly. Put carrots in a single layer into the air fryer. Cook for 10 mins or until soft, stirring once.

3. Move cooked carrots to a wide bowl. Add the balsamic glaze and the butter, and then toss to coat again. Now Sprinkle pepper before serving.

25.   Air-Fried Brussels Sprouts

Preparation Time: 10min | Serving: 2 | Difficulty: Easy

Nutritional Info: Calories: 78kcal | Fat: 7g | Carb: 28g | Protien: 4g

Ingredients

- Brussels sprouts, 1 pound

- Vegetable oil, 2 tablespoons

- Salt, ½ teaspoon Black pepper, ¼ teaspoon

- Mango nectar, 1/2 cup

- Rice vinegar, ¼ cup

- Brown sugar, ¼ cup

- Soy sauce, 1 tablespoon

- Cornstarch, 2 teaspoons

- Fish sauce, 1½ teaspoons

- Chile sauce, 1 teaspoon

Steps for preparation

1. Preheat the air fryer to about 375°F. In a large bowl, add oil, salt and pepper with Brussels sprouts. Place

the Brussels sprouts in a single layer in the air fryer basket.

2. Now Cook for 10-12 mins or until sprouts are soft and then stirring once.

3. For the sauce, mix mango nectar, rice vinegar, brown sugar, soya sauce, cornstarch, fish sauce and chili sauce in a shallow saucepan. Cook and mix until thickened. Now Cook and stir for 2 more mins.

4. Serve the sauce.

26. Air-Fryer Avocado Fries

Preparation Time: 15min | Serving: 2 | Difficulty: Easy

Nutritional Info: Calories: 267kcal | Fat: 8g | Carb: 23g | Protien: 5g

Ingredients

- All-purpose flour, ½ cup
- Black pepper, 1/2 teaspoons
- Eggs, 2
- Water, 1 tablespoon
- Bread crumbs (pano), ½ cup
- Avocados, 2 Cooking spray, as needed
- Kosher salt, ¼ teaspoon
- No-salted ketchup, ¼ cup
- Mayonnaise canola, 2 tablespoons
- Apple cider vinegar, 2 teaspoons
- Sriracha chili sauce, 1 tablespoon

Steps for preparation

1. Stir flour and pepper together in a shallow bowl.

2. Beat the eggs and water in a second shallow bowl. Put the panko in a third small bowl. Dredge the avocado wedges in flour, shaking the excess. Dip in the egg mixture. Coat the avocado wedges with the cooking spray.

3. Place the avocado wedges in the air fryer and cook at about 400°F till golden, 7-8 mins, turning the avocado wedges through the cooking process. Remove from the air fryer, season with salt.

4. When the avocado wedges are cooked, whisk together ketchup, mayonnaise, vinegar and the Sriracha in a small cup. To serve, put the 4 avocado fries on every plate with the 2 tablespoons of sauce.

27. Egg Rolls Air Fried

Preparation Time: 5min | Serving: 9 | Difficulty: Easy

Nutritional   Info: Calories: 78kcal | Fat: 6g | Carb:

7g | Protien: 1g

Ingredients

- Wrappers for egg roll, 6

- Shredded cabbage, 3 cups

- Shredded carrot, 1/4 cup

- Sesame oil, 1.5 teaspoon

- Grated ginger, 2 teaspoons

- Garlic clove, 1

- Soy sauce, 1 teaspoon

- Black pepper, 1/4 teaspoon

- Green onions, 2 Olive oil, 1 teaspoon

Steps for preparation

1. Preheat the frying pan over medium heat for few

   minutes. Add sesame oil, ginger, garlic, cabbage

   and shredded carrot.

2. Now Cook for 2 to 3 mins or till the cabbage has wilted. Add green onions, soya sauce and black pepper. Now stir and then remove the heat.

3. Assemble all the egg rolls. Brush with olive oil the egg rolls.

4. Brush with the olive fryer basket. Put egg rolls in the basket, seam side down.

5. And cook for 7 mins at about 360F. Flip and then again cook for 2 minutes.

28.   Stuffed Mushrooms Air Fried

Preparation Time: 15min | Serving: 4 | Difficulty: Easy

Nutritional   Info: Calories: 44kcal | Fat: 4g | Carb: 2g | Protien: 2g

Ingredients

- Large mushrooms, 16

- Salted butter, 1 tablespoon

- Garlic cloves, 2

- Onion minced, ½ cup

- Cream cheese, 4 oz

- Thyme leaves, ¼ teaspoon

- Worcestershire sauce, 1 teaspoon

- Fresh chopped parsley, 1 tablespoon

- Parmesan cheese, ¼ cup

- Pepper, I pinch

Steps for preparation

1. Clean the mushrooms and cut the stems. Finely dice the stems.

2. In a shallow pan, combine the stems, garlic, onions and butter. Cook till the onions are soft. Cool the mixture.

3. Mix onion paste with cream cheese, thyme, Worcestershire, parsley, pepper and 3 tablespoons of parmesan cheese.

4. Fill the mushroom caps with the cream cheese, and then sprinkle parmesan cheese over the top.

5. Put the ready caps in the air fryer and then cook at about 380°F for 7-9 mins.

29.   Air Fryer Squash

Preparation Time: 5min | Serving: 2 | Difficulty: Easy

Nutritional   Info: Calories: 39kcal | Fat: 4g | Carb:

2g | Protien: 1g

Ingredients

- Medium-sized summer squash, 1

- Italian seasoning, ½ teaspoon

- Olive oil, 1 tablespoon

- Salt & pepper, as per taste

Steps for preparation

1. Slice the courgettis into 1/2" slices.

2. Add the olive oil and the seasonings.

3. Preheat the air fryer to about 400°F.

4. Put squash in the air fryer and then cook for 6-7 mins

    or until soft and crisp. Now Cook 2 mins longer if you

    want a softer squash.

CHAPTER 5:

Dessert Recipes

Everyone loves a desert after a good meal, so we have not ignored this section in our book. Just go through this chapter, and you will be amazed to see a whole bunch of desert recipes you can easily make in your Air Fryer.

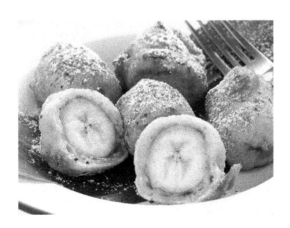

30. Air Fryer Sticks Donut

Preparation Time: 20min | Serving: 8 | Difficulty: Easy

Nutritional Info: Calories: 266kcal | Fat: 11.8g | Carb: 37.6g | Protien: 2.2g

Ingredients

- Crescent roll dough, 8 ounces

- Butter, melted, ¼ cup

- White sugar, ½ cup

- The ground cinnamon, 2 teaspoons

- Fruit jam, ½ cup

Steps for preparation

1. Flatten the crescent-shaped dough and then mold it into an 8-inch by 12-inch rectangle.

2. Sauté inside the air fryer, about four to five minutes, until the sides have become golden brown.

3. Pour a solution of sugar and cinnamon into a bowl and use a spoon to mix the ingredients, cut the

doughnut sticks, and then roll them in cinnamon-

sugar to cover.

4. Dip the doughnuts in the strawberry preserve and

enjoy.

31.   Air Fryer Chocolate Cake

Preparation Time: 10min | Serving: 4 | Difficulty: Easy

Nutritional Info: Calories: 214kcal | Fat: 11.7g | Carb: 25.5g | Protien: 3.2g

Ingredients

- Cooking oil
- White sugar, ¼ cup
- Butter, softened, 3 ½ tablespoons
- Egg, 1
- Apricot jam, 1 tablespoon
- All-purpose flour, 6 tablespoons
- Cocoa powder, 1 tablespoon
- Salt, to taste

Steps for preparation

1. Preheat the air fryer at 350F.
2. Beat egg and jam together. To ensure proper mixing, sift the flour, the cocoa powder, and the salt together.

3. Now fill any mold of your choice with this batter.

4. Bake inside the air fryer for about 4 minutes or until edges begin to turn golden brown. If the toothpick added into the cake comes out clean, then remove it from the air fryer and allow it to cool in the pan for a total of 5 minutes.

32. Air Fryer Cookie Fries Shortbread

Preparation Time: 20min | Serving: 20 | Difficulty: Easy

Nutritional Info: Calories: 88kcal | Fat: 4.1g | Carb: 12g | Protien: 0.7g

Ingredients

- All-purpose flour, 1 ¼ cups

- White sugar, 3 tablespoons

- Butter, ½ cup

- Strawberry jam, ⅓ cup

- Lemon curd, ⅓ cup

Steps for preparation

1. Dissolve sugar and the flour in a small bowl and knead for several minutes to combine into a stiff dough.

2. Take one-quarter of the dough. Stretch it out to a thickness of 1/4 inch. Parts and carve into one -a-half to two-inch "fries." Sprinkle some sugar on top.

3. Using a fine strainer, pulse in a bit of ground chipotle for an extra spicy finish. Beat the cream cheese to make it somewhat thicker to build a dip-able consistency for "mustard" sauce.

4. Now place the dough into the air fryer and bake for about 10 minutes at 350F.

5. When done, take out and let to cool for 5 minutes and serve.

33. Air Fryer Easy French Toast Sticks

Preparation Time: 10min | Serving: 2 | Difficulty: Easy

Nutritional Info: Calories: 232kcal | Fat: 7.4g | Carb: 60g

protein: 10 g

Ingredients

- Slightly stale, 4 slices

- Parchment paper

- Eggs, beaten, 2

- Milk, ¼ cup

- Vanilla extract, 1 teaspoon

- Cinnamon, 1 teaspoon

Steps for preparation

1. Cut every slice of the bread into large slices around 1/3/4 inch thick

2. Preheat the air fryer to 350F.

3. Add cinnamon, nutmeg, and the milk into the egg bowl good blended.

4. Place bread pieces in the egg mixture, ensuring sure they are coated with the egg mixture on both sides.

5. Place the coated bread pieces into the air fryer and back for 5 minutes from each side at 250F.

34. Air Fryer Jelly S'mores & Peanut Butter

Preparation Time: 5min | Serving: 2 | Difficulty: Easy

Nutritional Info: Calories: 249kcal | Fat: 8.2g | Carb: 41.2g | Protien: 3.9g

Ingredients

- Chocolate-topped with peanut butter, 1 cup
- Chocolate graham, 2
- Raspberry jam, 1 teaspoon
- Large marshmallow, 1

Steps for preparation

1. Spread 2 peanut-butter-crowded graham crackers with the raspberry jam. Finish off with a layer of marshmallow icing. Put in the air fryer carefully.

2. Now cook in the air fryer at 350F for 10 minutes. Take them out and enjoy.

35. Air Fryer Cookie Bites Chocolate Chip

Preparation Time: 10min | Serving: 16 | Difficulty: Easy

Nutritional Info: Calories: 188kcal | Fat: 10.4g | Carb: 23.6g | Protien: 2g

Ingredients

- White sugar, ¼ cup

- Baking soda, ½ teaspoon

- Salt, ½ teaspoon

- Egg, 1

- Vanilla extract, 1 ½ teaspoon

- All-purpose flour, 1 ⅓ cups

- Chocolate chips, 1 cup

- Finely sliced pecans, grilled, ⅓ cup

Steps for preparation

1. Extract paper from a roll or sheet using a cookie cutter to match the size of the air fryer's basket.

2. Beat the butter until moist and fluffy, then transfer it to the confectioners' bowl and beat until mixed. Add the confectioners' sugar and begin to beat until smooth, then raise the speed to fast and beat for an additional thirty seconds. Combine brown sugar, vinegar, baking soda, and the salt until light and creamy; beat on the medium for two minutes, sometimes scraping the bowl. Beat until mixed, then incorporate the egg and the vanilla until light and fluffy.

3. Place dough by the teaspoons into a parchment-lined baking dish spaced 1 inch apart. Be careful as you put lower the parchment into the air fryer.

4. Now cook in an air fryer at a temperature of 350F for 10 minutes.

5. Check the cooking texture and if you need more hard texture, then cook for some more time but make sure not to overcook.

36. Air Fryer Donut Bites Apple Cider

Preparation Time: 10min | Serving: 20 | Difficulty: Easy

Nutritional Info: Calories: 132kcal | Fat: 2.6g | Carb: 30g | Protien: 1.7g

Ingredients

- All-purpose flour, 2 ¼ cups

- White sugar, 3 tablespoons

- Baking powder, 4 teaspoons

- Apple pie spice, 1 ½ teaspoon

- Salt, ½ teaspoon

- Apple sauce, 4 ounces

- Apple cider, ½ cup Unsalted butter, ¼ cup

- Egg, 1 large Apple cider vinegar, 1 teaspoon

- Powdered sugar, 2 cups

- Apple pie spice, ½ teaspoon

Steps for preparation

1. Put flour, sugar, baking powder, and spices in a big bowl and mix thoroughly.

2. In a shallow bowl, mix ¼ cup of apple sauce, ⅓ cup of sparkling apple cider, a half cup of butter, and 2 teaspoons of vinegar; then blend well. Start by mixing in the brittle ingredients and insert the liquids into the mixture.

3. Now cook in the air fryer for 10 minutes at 350F.

4. Once the liquid is absorbed, increase heat to 375 degrees. And cook for 6 more minutes. Return the donut to the plate. Allow them to cool.

5. Whisk together apple juice and caramel extract for creating a smooth glaze.

6. Allow each donut to soak up a little bit of the coating and then roll this in the glaze; therefore, both sides are coated.

37.   Air Fryer Scones Strawberry

Preparation Time: 5min | Serving: 4 | Difficulty: Easy

Nutritional Info: Calories: 361kcal | Fat: 12g | Carb: 55g | Protien: 7g

Ingredients

- Flour, 225 g

- Butter, 50 g

- Caster Sugar, 50 g

- Milk, 60 ml

- Vanilla Essence

- Fresh Strawberries, 50 g

- Whipped Cream, 4 tablespoons

- Strawberry Jam, 1 tablespoon

Steps for preparation

1. Place the flour, the butter, and the sugar into the bowl and add them together until the sugar is thoroughly incorporated. Finally, mix vanilla to

produce a smooth mixture, somewhat sticky dough.

2. Divide into 4 similar portions and roll each into a disc. Flatten each portion and make four balls in the form of scones.

3. Carefully put these ball shapes in the air fryer and cook at 375F for 10 minutes.

38. **Pudding Berry Bread**

Preparation Time: 10min | Serving: 4 | Difficulty: Easy

Nutritional Info: Calories: 239kcal | Fat: 13g | Carb: 26g | Protien: 6g

Ingredients

- Cream, ½ cup

- Milk, ½ cup

- Eggs, 2

- Sugar granulated, 3 tablespoons

- Lemon Extract, ½ teaspoon

- Brioche cubed, 3 slices

- Raspberries, ½ cup

- Blueberries, ⅓ cup

- Butter Powdered sugar, 1 teaspoon

- Maple syrup

Steps for preparation

1. Coat a pan with butter and then place it in an air fryer basket. Cut the loaf into tiny cubes. Whisk the

eggs, the sugar and the lemon zest together in a bowl. Using a mixer, mix till they are well-blended to produce soft-serve ice cream.

2. Bake on a single sheet. For making jam, spread a handful of blueberries on the brioche. Put a second brioche on top of it and sprinkle some fruit over the top.

3. Then, coat the brioche with the custard.

4. Use a spatula to press both of the brioches onto the custard to ensure it gets soaked. Just let the custard mixture sit for ten minutes.

5. To set up the baking tray, put it inside the air fryer bake basket for about 10 minutes at 350F.

39. Air Fryer Cake Egg & Chocolate

Preparation Time: 10min | Serving: 4 | Difficulty: Easy

Nutritional Info: Calories: 483kcal | Fat: 33g | Carb: 43g | Protien: 5g

Ingredients

- Butter, 7 tablespoons
- Chocolate chips, 1 c
- Eggs, 2
- Sugar, 3.5 tablespoon
- Flour, 1.5 tablespoon

Steps for preparation

1. Melt chocolate and then sugar. Put into the boiling water inside a pot for 30 seconds.

2. Beat the sugar with an electric mixer until light and frothy. Now whisk the egg combination till the mixture is smooth.

3. Now, blend until smooth.

4. Draw 4 identical portions of batter into 4 clean ramekins.

5. Now cook them in the air fryer for about 10 minutes on 350F.

40. Air Fryer Peach Muffins

Preparation Time: 10min | Serving: 6 | Difficulty: Easy

Nutritional Info: Calories: 196kcal | Fat: 7g | Carb: 29g | Protien: 3g

Ingredients

- Plain flour, 1 cup 137g

- Baking powder, 1 teaspoon

- Peach zest, 1/2 teaspoon

- Salt, 1/8 teaspoon

- Vegetable oil, 2.5 tablespoons

- Sugar, 1/3 cup 50g

- Milk, 1/3 cup 90ml

- Egg, 1

- Vanilla essence, 1/2 teaspoon

- Peach, 1/2 cup 80g

- Raw vanilla sugar, 1/2 tablespoon

Steps for preparation

1. Insert a paper liner into a muffin cup.

2. Combine the flour, baking powder and salt in a big bowl.

3. Add the oil, cream, peach, vanilla and sugar into the bowl and mix until it is well blended.

4. Split the batter equally among the muffin cups, blend the muffin dough, and spread it among the wholes.

5. Line a muffin tray with aluminum foil, put it into the air fryer, and then bake for 12 minutes.

6. The muffins should be set for a few minutes on the baking sheet before removing them from the air fryer.

41.   **Air Fryer Suhoogar Daunts**

Preparation Time: 5min | Serving: 8 | Difficulty: Easy

Nutritional   Info: Calories: 135kcal | Fat: 3g | Carb: 16g | Protien: 1g

Ingredients

- Pillsbury Biscuits, 1 Cane

- Sugar, 1/2 Cup

- Cinnamon, 1/2 tablespoon

- Butter, 5 tablespoons

Steps for preparation

1. Whisk the cinnamon and the sugar together inside a bowl when mixed.

2. Open the can of the biscuits and use a can-opener to cut the hole in the middle of the cane.

3. Place the butter in a small saucepan and heat over medium flame.

4. Now mash the biscuits, add some melted butter to make a dough, and make a round shape. Now put

4-5 rounds in your air fryer and bake at 375F for 15 minutes.

5. Once baking is done, take them out and Cover the doughnuts with some molten butter using the silicone pastry brush. Next, you should add cinnamon-sugar at and use a spoon to spread it properly

CHAPTER 6:

Snacks And Treat Recipes

S ay goodbye to your hunger by enjoying hundreds of easy-to-make snacks and treat recipes mention in this chapter.

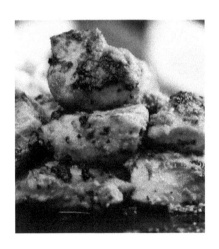

42. Zucchini, Corn And Haloumi Fritters In An Air Fryer

Preparation Time: 12min | Serving: 3 | Difficulty: Easy

Nutritional Info: Calories: 119kcal | Fat: 4g | Carb: 9g | Protien: 3g

Ingredients

- Medium zucchini, 2

- Block halloumi, 225g

- Frozen corn kernels, 150g

- Eggs, 2

- Flour, 100g

- Fresh oregano leaves, 3 teaspoons

- Natural yogurt, to serve

- Fresh oregano, to serve

Steps for preparation

1. Squeeze remaining moisture from zucchini with your hands. Put the zucchini in a mixing bowl. Combine the halloumi and the corn in a mixing

cup. To mix, stir all together. Make a well in the middle of the mixture and add egg, flour, and oregano. Season with salt and pepper and mix until well blended.

2. Preheat air fryer to 200F. Place tablespoons of zucchini mixture on a rack of an air fryer. Cook for about 8 minutes, or until the bacon is crisp and golden. Place on a tray.

3. Serve the warm patties on a tray, in a small bowl, place yogurt. Serve with the extra oregano on it.

43.   Corn In An Air Fryer

Preparation Time: 7min | Serving: 2 | Difficulty: Easy

Nutritional Info: Calories: 117kcal | Fat: 2g | Carb: 8g | Protien: 2g

Ingredients

- Ear corn, 4

- Olive oil, 2 tablespoons

- Salt, 1 teaspoon

- Ground paprika, 1 teaspoon

Steps for preparation

1. Preheat air fryer to about 400F.

2. Brush each of the ear corn with olive oil and season with salt and paprika powder.

3. Place corn in an air fryer on a single sheet.

4. Cook for 20 mins, turning halfway through, till the kernels are soft golden brown.

5. Sprinkle with parsley and nutritional yeast.

44. Roasted Edamame In Air Fryer

Preparation Time: 12min | Serving: 2 | Difficulty: Easy

Nutritional Info: Calories: 74kcal | Fat: 1g | Carb: 4g | Protien: 6g

Ingredients

- Edamame, 2 cups
- Olive oil spray
- Garlic salt

Steps for preparation

1. Put edamame in an air fryer basket.
2. Coat with the olive oil spray and the garlic salt to taste.
3. Air fry at 390°F for 10 mins.
4. If desired, stir halfway through cooking time. Air fry for extra 5 mins for crispy flavor.
5. Serve.

45. Tofu In An Air Fryer

Preparation Time: 10min | Serving: 2 | Difficulty: Easy

Nutritional Info: Calories: 98kcal | Fat: 2g | Carb: 4g | Protien: 2g

Ingredients

- Block tofu, 1 16-oz

- Sesame oil, 2 tablespoons

- Garlic powder, 1 teaspoon

- Onion powder, 1 teaspoon

- Salt, 1/4 teaspoon

Steps for preparation

1. Slice Tofu into the small, even cubes.

2. Put tofu cubes on a plate lined with paper towels to push out as much water as possible.

3. Toss tofu cubes with sesame oil, garlic powder, onion powder, and salt until the tofu has been pressed. Allow at least 15 mins for it to marinate.

4. Preheat air fryer to 375F.

5. Place tofu cubes in a single layer in an air fryer basket.

6. Now Cook for about 10 -12 mins, tossing halfway through, for the tofu that is golden on the outside yet fluffy on the inside. Now Cooked for about 14 to 15 mins.

46.   Seasoned Pretzels In Air Fryer

Preparation Time: 7min | Serving: 2 | Difficulty: Easy

Nutritional Info: Calories: 148kcal | Fat: 3g | Carb: 18g | Protien: 4g

Ingredients

- Regular Pretzels, 8oz

- Ranch Seasoning, 1 Packet

- Garlic Powder, ¼ tablespoon

- Olive Oil Spray

Steps for preparation

1. Spray air fryer basket with olive oil, then cover with aluminum foil.

2. Put the pretzels in a basket, sprinkle with the ranch seasoning and the garlic powder.

3. Spray a few coats of olive oil on pretzels.

4. Cook for about 3 mins at 350°F in an air fryer.

5. Remove pretzels with caution, brush with olive oil, then blend.

6. Cook for a total of 3 minutes more.

7. Remove pretzels with caution, brush with olive oil spray, then blend.

8. Cook for another 2 minutes, just until pretzels are soft and crispy.

47. Parmesan Zucchini Crisps In Air Fryer

Preparation Time: 15min | Serving: 2 | Difficulty: Easy

Nutritional Info: Calories: 124kcal | Fat: 7g | Carb: 4g | Protien: 11g

Ingredients

- Medium zucchini sliced into ¼ inch thick rounds, 1
- Grated parmesan cheese, ½ cup

Steps for preparation

1. Put zucchini rounds in a single sheet in an air fryer. Cover the surface of each round with a thin layer of parmesan cheese.

2. Preheat air fryer to 370°F. Now Cook rounds for 12 mins, or until the cheese is golden brown. Let rounds cool for few minutes to allow the cheese to be crisp more.

3. Toss with your preferred dipping sauce and serve...

48.   **Brats In Air Fryer**

Preparation Time: 7min | Serving: 2 | Difficulty: Easy

Nutritional   Info: Calories: 57kcal | Fat: 5g | Carb:

2g | Protien: 12g

Ingredients

- Uncooked brats, 1 pack

Steps for preparation

1. Place the raw brats in the air fryer basket.

2. Air fry brats for 12-15 mins at 350°F, turning halfway through. Now They are over until their internal temperature reaches 160F.

3. Remove brats from the air fryer basket with the tongs and put them aside for 5 minutes to rest.

49. Stuffed Mushrooms In Air Fryer

Preparation Time: 10min | Serving: 2 | Difficulty: Easy

Nutritional Info: Calories: 86kcal | Fat: 8g | Carb: 3g | Protien: 2g

Ingredients

- Mushrooms, 16 oz

- Cream Cheese, 6 oz

- Sour Cream, 3 tablespoons

- Shredded Cheddar Cheese, 1/4 cup

- Garlic Powder, ½ tablespoon

- Salt, ½ tablespoon

- Dash of Pepper

- Chopped Chives for topping

- Oil Spray

Steps for preparation

1. Remove dirt from mushrooms with a wet paper towel. Remove mushroom caps' stems by popping them off.

2. In a mixing bowl, combine the cream cheese, sour cream, garlic powder, salt, and pepper. Fill mushroom caps "well" with the mixture. Top with the shredded cheddar cheese and the chives on each.

3. To save the air fryer from sticking, coat with the oil spray. Fill the basket with a single layer of mushrooms. Preheat the oven to 370°F and cook for about 8-10 mins. Allow cooling for few minutes before serving.

50. Sweet Carrot Fries In Air Fryer

Preparation Time: 5min | Serving: 1 | Difficulty: Easy

Nutritional Info: Calories: 20kcal | Fat: 1g | Carb: 4g | Protien: 1g

Ingredients

- Medium carrots, 2

- Olive oil, 1 tablespoon

- Lemon herb seasoning, 2 tablespoons

Steps for preparation

1. Slice Carrots into "French fry" shaped pieces.

2. In mixing cup, blend vegetables, oil, and seasoning.

3. Toss carrots until finely coated. Now Air fries at about 350°F for 15 minutes, shaking halfway through.

CHAPTER 7:

Frequently Asked Questions About Most Common Issues With The Air Fryer!

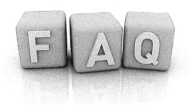

This section of the book contains some common yet frequently asked questions about the air fryer's issues. In this section, you will learn how to deal with these issues and get the most out of your machine.

1.1 Common Issues With An Air Fryer And Their Solutions

1. My Air fryer Is not turning on:

This is the most frequently asked question. If you face the same problem, first check that you have properly inserted the power outlet's power cord. Next, make sure that the power wire is not damaged (before checking 1ˢᵗ unplug your Air fryer from the main power outlet).

2. My Air fryer releases smoke some time when cooking food?

Well, it is not a big issue sometimes when you cook fatty food in the air fryer it produces some smoke.

Note: if the smoke is blue, then it's a clear indication that there is an electrical fault in your machine. in this case, never use the machine and contact the manufacturer's recommended dealer for assistance.

3. My Air fryer does not cook crispy food?

Well, the main reason is that food is not being properly cooked in your machine, there is a various reason which causes this issue:

- Too much food in the air fryer basket
- You have not pre-heated the machine before putting food inside the basket.
- The drawer containing the air fryer's basket is not properly closed.
- Temperature is not properly set
- You have not shuffled the food in between the cooking process.

4. My Air fryer Produces noise?

It is normal because the machine uses air as a medium to transfer the heat to your food, and the fan is rotating at high speed; also, the fan inside electrical appliances is responsible for reducing the internal temperature of machines; hence the sound may go up to 65 decibels.

5. My air fryer overcooks the food

It has been observed that most of the times the cooking duration mentioned in recipes is not 10% correct. Also, environmental factors greatly affect the time needed to cook the food; hence, it is necessary to check the food while cooking to avoid this issue.

6. My food always has a dry texture

Most people think that an air fryer does not need oil to cook the food. You can indeed cook the food in an air fryer without using oil, but some foods need oil while cooking them, so make sure you follow the proper recipe.

7. My machine throws out some quantity of food while cooking

When you put some light weight food in the air fryer, it mostly happens with bread crumbs, so it is advised to use a rack of iron over the food, which has this kind of texture and is light in weight.

8. After using it a few times, my air fryer produces the smell

Well, it happens when you cook the food and do not properly clean the basket and drawer. When we cook food, some amount of fat and leftover pieces of food stick to the fryer's sidewalls and make deposits in the drawer and basket of the air fryer. Hence it is highly recommended to wash after every single use the basket and drawer of your machine.

Note: some models may not have a detachable drawer, so cleaning must follow the manufacturer's manual.

9. My device did not switch off

In some models, there is the switch at the bottom which some time stuck, so make sure you place the machine on a flat surface, and there must be some space between the machine bottom and surface on which it is placed

So, these are some common issues with an air fryer and people mostly asked about them, so if you face any of them, find the solution here in this section of the book.

If you face any other issue, then 1st go through the manufacturer's manual; if you do not find the solution, contact the authorized dealer.

Note: never try to open the machine by yourself because it has electrical components; hence there is always a hazard of electric shock.

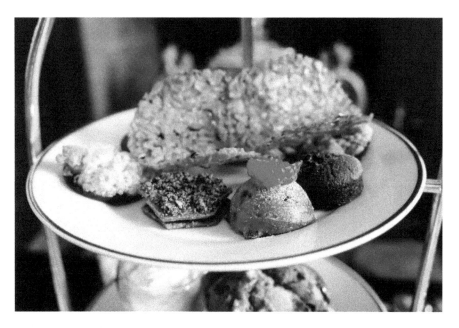

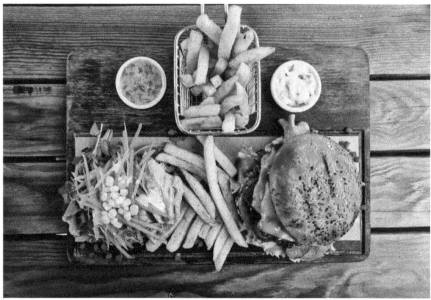

Conclusion

You may have noticed that now a days many people talk about healthy life style and prefer the food which offers health benefits. Conventionally people prefer boiled foods because it involves less or no amount of oil. The excess use of oil and fat build up cholesterol levels and hence cause various disease. But we know that not every food can be cooked using the boiling method.

Air fryer is a perfect alternative hence we have provided our user a proper and comprehensive guide that can easily be followed and learn how to use air fryer for cooking food.

We have provided a brief guide which you can be followed to understand how an air fryer works and how to properly handle it with safety, we have provided hundreds of recipes in this book which are easy to make and you will love them. For your ease we have divided them in sections so you don't have to go through the whole book to find out your favorite recipes. For your ease we have divided this book in 5 sections (Meat, Vegetables, Sea Food, Desert and Snacks) just go through each section and you will love to have your favorite recipe.

Lightning Source UK Ltd.
Milton Keynes UK
UKHW020754230421
382490UK00005B/92